MORDEN GUIDE TO NURTURING YOUR KIDS

A panacea to abuse, neglect, abandonment, violent and abduction which many children in America live with

Dr. R. Spock

Copyright@2021 R. Spock

INTRODUCTION	**4**
CHAPTER ONE	**10**
SECURING YOUR KID	10
SUPPORTING YOUR KID'S ADVANCEMENT FROM 6 TO 9 MONTHS	12
WHAT DEVELOPMENT LOOKS LIKE IN REGULAR DAY TO DAY EXISTENCE?	13
CONNECTIONS ARE THE ESTABLISHMENT OF A YOUNGSTER'S SOUND TURN OF EVENTS	14
DIAGRAMMING YOUR YOUNGSTER'S SOLID TURN OF EVENTS	14
CHAPTER TWO	**16**
WHAT'S GOING ON: WHAT YOU CAN DO: QUESTIONS TO ASK YOURSELF:	16
FIVE CHARACTERISTICS TO SUPPORT IN A KID	18
CHAPTER 3	**30**
EIGHT DIFFERENT WAYS TO SUPPORT A KID'S SPIRIT	30
BE A SORTER OF THEIR KNOT.	31
CAUSE THEM TO FEEL LIKE THE MAIN INDIVIDUAL ON THE PLANET.	32
THE ADVANTAGES OF THE CONSTRUCTION JOB	40
WHEN GIVING CONSTRUCTION, YOUR KIDS:	40
CHAPTER 4	**49**
THE SUSTAINING GUARDIAN	51
PROTECT YOUR YOUNGSTERS, REGARDLESS!	55
THERE ARE TWO KINDS OF YOUTH ENCOUNTERS	56
WHAT IS A SUPPORTING RELATIONSHIP AND HOW TO LOOK AFTER IT?	59
WHAT IS SUPPORTING?	60
CHARACTER AND GOOD KNOWLEDGE, NURTURING	68

SEVEN STRAIGHTFORWARD REGARD BUILDING NURTURING PRACTICES	70
CHAPTER 5	**76**
CONCLUSION	**76**

Introduction

Nurturing implies more than giving your kid food, haven and attire. It is tied in with building a solid and forceful enthusiastic relationship (connection) among you and your kid. It implies being the individual your kid can depend on for solace whether he is a fastidious baby or a little child having a fit. It implies being your youngster's protected base. The individual he can go to for affection, wellbeing and security as he investigates the enormous world around him.

Examination shows that when you sustain your youngster, your kid is bound to be solid, fruitful in school, ready to coexist with different kids, and better ready to deal with pressure.

However, significant as it seems to be, sustaining isn't in every case simple. For instance, in some cases when your infant is crying, you don't have the foggiest idea why and nothing you do solaces him. Each parent has that experience, feeling powerless and dubious on occasion. In any case, hold tight. Attempt to remain quiet. Tell your infant you love him and that together you will sort it out. Since you will—yet it requires some serious energy.

The Public Asset Place for Local area Based Youngster Misuse Counteraction has recognized five defensive factors that influence the prosperity of kids and families. Supporting is recorded as one of the defensive elements and when present, it can expand the wellbeing and prosperity of youngsters and families.

The Merriam-Webster word reference characterizes the word support as "preparing or childhood,""something that feeds." The word sustain comes from the Latin word "nurture" which intends to nurture, feed and to advance development. Words that have a comparative importance to the word sustain incorporate empower, hatch, further and advance. All individuals should be sustained and supporting necessities to start before birth and proceed all through life.

There are numerous ways that grown-ups sustain. Four deliberate ways that a parent or guardian can sustain kids include:

Practice sympathy - Compassion necessitates that you notice another's activities, perceive the connected inclination that they are having and afterward express it such that shows that you comprehend. Therapist Alfred Adler clarified it along these lines; Sympathy is "seeing with the eyes of another, tuning in with the ears of another and feeling with the core of another." This can be troublesome on the off chance that you have not experienced compassion yourself. Start by noticing an inclination in a kid, give the inclination a name and afterward utilizing the name of the inclination in a "you" message. "You should be disappointed at not having the option to fit the unique piece around there.""You presumably wish that your companions would have gone to bat for you.""You are furious in light of the fact that Joey took your toy and broke it."

Build up schedules - Youngsters need plans and rely upon grown-ups in their life to give construction to them. You can support your youngster by giving standard dinner, play, study and sleep time schedules. By giving a timetable your kid learns consistency through redundancy, security through understanding what will occur straightaway and some authority over their current circumstance. A normal routine empowers youngsters to lessen nervousness by realizing what is coming straightaway.

Utilize positive touch - We as a whole have a requirement for human touch. A positive touch is an embrace, pat, delicate tickle or delicate poke. Normal warm and delicate contacts can assist youngsters with building up a sound ability to be self aware and can add to positive mental health. Positive touch can help a kid with recapturing control when they are being diverted after misconduct.
Protect kids from hurt - Kids who are little need to have a sense of security in their own homes, childcare, in their

networks and in the bigger world around them. Give cutoff points to the kids in your day to day existence by giving a protected climate. Pick kid care suppliers cautiously. Use vehicle seats, infant doors and other endorsed hardware for small kids. Investigate open air play zones for likely dangers and have decides for inside play that take into consideration learning while at the same time limiting unsatisfactory exercises for little children and preschoolers.

Discussion about expected risks without alarming your kids

Family amicable data is accessible from Safe Children, an association that is committed to furnishing guardians and parental figures with reasonable assets to shield kids from wounds.

Nurturing and providing care can be an unpleasant occupation that requires some investment and penance. It is critical to set an illustration of sustaining for youngsters by supporting yourself. Put away an ideal opportunity to benefit you. At the point when grown-ups sustain themselves by having their own requirements met, they are more ready to address the issues of their kids. The four ideas expressed above additionally apply to sustaining yourself; perceive and name your sentiments, adhere to a timetable, give and get delicate touch and shield yourself from things that could hurt you.

Sustaining doesn't fall into place for all grown-ups and supporting practices can be learned. Kids who are supported figure out how to treat themselves, others and their current circumstance in a sustaining way. Michigan State College Expansion offers projects and occasions that can help with acquiring new supporting abilities or enhancing those you as of now have.

Chapter One
Securing Your Kid

This may appear glaringly evident; obviously every parent needs to shield their kids from hurt." Yet "hurt" isn't in every case simple to see—in any event, when it is directly before your eyes. Since youngsters develop and change so rapidly, the opportunities for hurt change as well. Yet, security leads won't ever change:

Shield your kid from hazardous individuals and spots

Shield your kid from sickness with inoculations and great cleanliness

Shield your kid from harms like recycled smoke and lead

Shield your kid from consumes by checking the temperature of shower water

Secure your home by having working smoke and carbon monoxide indicators

Alternate approaches to secure your kid will change as she creates. For instance, the standard of taking care of newborn children on their backs ("Back to Rest") doesn't matter to babies who turn over and move around the bunk in their rest. The sort of vehicle seat you need and its situation in the vehicle additionally changes as your kid develops.

In this Guide, you will find out about ways you can secure your youngster during her first long stretches of life. It doesn't cover everything—no guide can. Yet, it can help you make the association between your kid's changing capacities and requirements, new possible wellsprings of mischief, and how your words and activities should change to keep her safe.

Infants appear on the scene pre-wired to learn, impart, and associate with you. You can see a baby conveying as you attempt to sort out what she needs dependent on her sounds (crying, snorting, cooing), articulations (shock, grinning, scowling), and body developments (whipping, kicking with satisfaction when she sees you).

Kids, even babies and little children, should be encircled by language consistently. How you speak with your baby appears to be unique than how you talk with your kid or four year old.

In this Guide, you will discover simple and functional approaches to speak with your youngster starting before birth and proceeding with completely through the pre-school years.

Supporting Your Kid's Advancement From 6 to 9 Months

Figure out how to support your infant's social, enthusiastic, scholarly, language, and engine improvement from 6 to 9 months.

Your relationship with your kid is the establishment of her sound turn of events.

Your youngster's advancement relies upon both the characteristics he was brought into the world with (nature), and what he encounters (support).

All spaces of advancement (social, enthusiastic, scholarly, language, and engine) are connected. Each relies upon, and impacts, the others.

What kid's insight, including how their folks react to them, shapes their advancement as they adjust to the world.

What Development Looks like in Regular day to day existence?

This model shows how all spaces of Reina's improvement are associated and how her mom's reaction upholds her sound turn of events.

Sophia is the mother of 9-month-old Reina. Sophia's dearest companion, Claudia, is coming into town to meet Reina interestingly. At the point when Claudia shows up, Reina will have nothing to do with her. Each time Claudia attempts to converse with or play with Reina she cries, dismisses, and sticks to Sophia. Sophia feels baffled and humiliated. While enticed to simply hand Reina to Claudia, she stops, and rather holds Reina on her lap and requests that Claudia sit close to them and read Reina's #2 book. Gradually Reina begins to take a gander at Claudia and shows expanding interest, before long Reina begins to creep off Sophia's lap to draw nearer to Claudia.

Reina's solid bond with her mom, the trust she shows as she sticks to her for security, and her dread of outsiders are generally indications of her social and passionate turn of events.

Connections are the establishment of a youngster's sound turn of events.

Her scholarly improvement empowers her to differentiate between who she knows and who she doesn't, and it assists her with finding a way ways to get the solace and assurance she needs. She utilizes her sounds (language improvement) and looks and signals (engine advancement) first to convey to Sophia that she is awkward and needs support. Later she utilizes them to impart that she is prepared to interface. Sophia's affectability to Reina's need to heat up gradually to new circumstances and individuals helps Reina feel cherished and secure, which will help her vibe more happy with meeting new individuals as she develops.

Diagramming Your Youngster's Solid Turn of events

The accompanying diagram depicts a considerable lot of the things your infant is learning somewhere in the range of 6 and 9 months and how you can deal with help your kid in every aspect of her turn of events. As you read, recall that youngsters create at their own speed and in their own particular manner. Understanding who your youngster is, the thing that her qualities are, and where she needs more help are fundamental for advancing her solid turn of events. In the event that you have questions in regards to your kid's turn of events, ask your pediatrician.

Chapter Two

What's going on: What you can do: Questions to ask yourself:

Infants this age are enormous communicators. They utilize numerous sounds, motions, and looks to impart what they want. Talk a ton with your infant. For instance, name and describe. "You're eating a major banana!" Give her chance to respond. How does your infant let you understand what she needs? What she's inclination and thinking?

Their activities are their interchanges. They might be beginning to assemble consonants and vowels to frame words like "dada" and "mama." Respond to her correspondences. Perceive how long you can keep a to and fro discussion going. For instance, she makes a sound, you mimic it, she makes another sound, thus on. What, all things considered; do you discover disappointing about understanding your child's correspondences? Why?

As her mind develops, your child will begin to copy others, particularly you. This prompts the advancement of heaps of new skills. Give your infant time to take in what you did and afterward duplicate you. Press a catch on the jack-in-the-container, at that point trust that your child will do it before you do it once more. This trains your child circumstances and logical results. Seeing that she can get things going forms her self-assurance and causes her need to take on new challenges. How to have you seen your infant impersonate?

Children this age can likewise utilize toys in more intricate manners. For instance, rather than simply holding a plastic cup, an infant this age may utilize it to pour water in the bathtub. Provide an assortment of safe toys for the shower—compartments, elastic toys, plastic shower books, and plastic spoons. These will urge your child to investigate and try different things with the various approaches to utilize objects. Obviously, never let your child be in the bath. What sort of play does your infant most appreciate? What does this inform you concerning her?

Their engine abilities permit them to get the thoughts in their mind going, for instance, getting the ball that moved away. Create a climate that is alright for investigation. Ensure just safe items are inside your child's grip and that anything she may use to pull herself dependent upon her feet is tough and secured down to the floor or divider. This sort of infant sealing of your home additionally will decrease clashes among you and your baby. What do you have to do to make your home more secure for your "little pilgrim?"

Five characteristics to support in a kid

Specialists say that fruitful, glad individuals—the individuals who do well in their picked vocations and structure fulfilling connections for the duration of their lives—will in general share certain characteristics. Furthermore, guardians can help support those critical attributes in their youngsters, in any event, when they're newborn children. Here's a glance at the best five characteristics your infant will require, as per kid improvement specialists, alongside certain ways you can begin your little one on the way to obtaining every one of these immeasurably significant resources.

1. Trust

An essential trust in others is the establishment on which any remaining attributes rest. Without this trademark, children face a difficult formative fight. She'll struggle building connections, feeling sure, and pushing ahead except if she can trust. Giving trust begins directly from the time your baby is conceived. You can bond with your child in a manner that ingrains in her a significant suspicion that all is well and good, a confidence on the planet—and eventually, in herself. In early stages, that implies reacting to her essential requirements. Feed her when she's ravenous. Rock her with she needs to be nestled, change her diaper when it's dirty. Yet in addition take advantage of your day by day communications by conversing with her, singing to her, and visually connecting. To make a truly protected inclination, present ceremonies, for example, perusing a story consistently before sleep time.

At the point when she's a baby, your youngster's necessities become more mind boggling. Obviously she should be taken care of, washed, and dealt with, yet she additionally needs you to see her scrawls and her square pinnacles. Recognizing her accomplishments may not appear as essential as, say, giving her supper, however it is. Attempt to focus on her signs and respond in like manner to her necessities.

Additionally focus on your infant's disposition. Not all kids are similar and your little one will confide in you more on the off chance that you tailor your activities to suit her character. A few infants, for instance, can take loads of incitement, while others appear to emit or close down when there's a lot going on. The more you show your child you comprehend her specific air, the more she'll feel that you're her ally.

2. Persistence

It's actual: Blessings will rain down on patient people. Children who learn tolerance can drive forward and are bound to succeed, says Claire Lerner, a youngster advancement expert with Zero to Three, a support bunch that centers around babies and little children. Showing a kid the nature of persistence can help ingrain in him a sensation of freedom and achievement.

Need to help your kid along? First recall this: Your infant is watching. On the off chance that you become violently unhinged when you face unpleasant traffic or a long queue, you'll set a helpless model. They're similar to wipes, taking everything in, says Jody Johnston Pawel, a parent instructor and creator of The Parent's Toolshop: The Widespread Outline for Building a Sound Family. Specialists call it demonstrating—make the best choice and your child is bound to follow. Become immediately exasperated when your baby spills his milk and you'll pass on one message; smoothly help him tidy it up and you'll show him something different totally.

Appending words to your little one's feelings additionally helps cultivate tolerance. Little children by and large can't say a ton, yet they see the greater part of what you advise them. So if your 18-month-old has a tantrum when he can't assemble his riddle, reveal to him you comprehend and recognize his dissatisfaction. Likewise, on the off chance that you end up going to blow a circuit, clarify how you feel as opposed to lashing out.

Little children don't have the very feeling of time that we do, which makes it much harder for them to show restraint. You can help by checking time in manners other than minutes and hours. For example, if your kid requests some juice when you're really busy washing dishes, instead of reacting with, "I'll get it quickly," have a go at saying "I'll get it when I'm done with these plates." Along these lines, he can watch your advancement and measure how before long he'll get his juice.

3. Obligation

To prevail throughout everyday life, says an expert, you need to realize how to make responsibilities and finish. It's something that even an infant can start to handle. Indeed, when your kid joyfully begins dropping her jug on the floor, hanging tight for you to get it, just to rehash this activity and once more, she's prepared to begin finding out about obligation. That is on the grounds that she has built up a simple comprehension of circumstances and logical results and the acknowledgment that there are ramifications to her activities.

In particular, that implies you can begin pondering infant size duties, such as giving her a spoon and requesting that she offer it to Father. As she develops more seasoned, you can make errands further developed, maybe requesting that she toss her socks in the hamper or stack her books. You'll make it all that amount more acceptable in the event that you additionally clarify the worth of each assignment. Yet, make a point to keep your clarifications brief to stay away from disarray; for instance, the hamper is "the place where grimy garments go to get perfect," and stacking books "makes it simple to discover what you need to peruse sometime later." She may not comprehend your clarifications from the start, however ultimately the thoughts will soak in.

Assisting with cleaning is, obviously, a helpful task. Yet, don't expect excessively. For a little child, getting more than three or four toys can be overpowering. Have a go at making it a game or singing a unique tidy up melody while you put the toys away.

Obviously, we're regularly hurried to the point that we deter our youngsters from tackling errands since it takes them excessively long. In case you're in a rush, pick a couple of key obligations—yet ensure you implement them.

4. Sympathy

Sympathy is critical to the advancement of an individual's social capability, says Phillips. To have effective connections, you need to realize how individuals are feeling and react properly. While even newborn children display a crude type of compassion, kids don't actually get equipped for imagining another's perspective until somewhere close to the ages of 3 and 6. Prior to at that point, they experience difficulty seeing the world from anybody's viewpoint however their own. At the point when a 2-year-old bops his companion on the head, he doesn't comprehend that it harms since he hasn't felt anything himself, says an expert

In any case, there's a ton you can do to assist a youngster with creating sympathy. Asking your baby, "How might you feel if that happened to you?" doesn't cut it, since he's so significantly egocentric. All things considered, disclose to him what his activities mean for other people. On the off chance that he nibbles his sibling, clarify that it harms and may cause a bungle. In the event that you see another kid with a cleaned knee, talk about how it should sting. Also, be prepared to offer those remarks again and again. This is one quality that needs a ton of rehashing before you can anticipate that it should take, says a therapist.

Be cautious about TV. In the event that you watch kid's shows wherein the characters beat up on each other, bring up how, all things considered, that would feel awful. While the contrast among the real world and dream is as yet hazy for your kid, you'll plant the seed of a significant exercise. Simultaneously, not all projects are hurtful, and some are even gainful.

Considerably more pivotal is your conduct as a parent. Do unto your youngster as you need your kid to do unto others, says Lerner. That implies focusing on his requirements and showing him that you regard his emotions. On the off chance that he tosses his colored pencils out of resentment, serenely demand that he help get them—yet reveal to him you comprehend that he's frantic as well.

5. Independence

By figuring out how to act autonomously, your youngster will grow up with a sufficient inward compass to understand what she needs and to make good decisions all alone. Maybe the best characteristic you can give to your kid - one that assists him with showing restraint, dependable, and independent—is the capacity to tackle issues. In the event that your 14-month-old is getting eager since she can't play with another kid's toy, recognize her misery, yet urge her to search for different arrangements, proposes an expert.

Help your kid break errands into little advances, and afterward let her lord each progression all alone. In the event that she can sort out some way to pull down her own towel, open the treat container, or spread jam on her toast, she'll feel more self-governing and sure about handling greater errands around the house.

You can likewise help construct independence by giving your youngster age-proper activities. At age 1, that may mean figuring out how to eat with a spoon, and after a year, putting on a baggy shirt. Make things as simple as could really be expected—purchase shoes with self-latches rather than bands, for instance—and be set up to help when fundamental. In the event that your little child frantically needs a treat, get her so she can open the bureau, get the bundle, and select one without anyone else.

Perhaps the most ideal ways for your kid to learn independence is by displaying your conduct. In case you're experiencing difficulty, say, gathering your new PC, converse with yourself so anyone can hear, strolling yourself through the means, so your kid can see you going through the way toward taking care of the issue.

While you're grinding away, remember to encourage your kid's uniqueness. Recall that it's critical to request and recognize her conclusions. In the event that you see her get a similar shirt over and over, say "That should be your top choice." When she's more established, you can empower more refined choices. When shopping, request your baby to choose a shirt from a decision from two. Ask whether she'd prefer play with her Frisbee or a ball.

Inconvenience is, instructing these characteristics can be tedious—allowing children to tackle their own issues requires some investment—and that is something guardians simply don't have. In any case, you'll help your kid more in the event that you oppose bouncing in and getting things done for her. That additional moment will pay off in the coming years.

A few children appear to be brought into the world with more confidence than others, however there's a great deal you can do to advance your kid's passionate prosperity — a more grounded ability to be self aware can make your youngster all the more genuinely strong when issues come his direction.

Accommodating your youngster's actual requirements (food, cover, apparel) is a genuinely direct matter. Attempting to accommodate your youngster's feelings can be trickier. Despite the fact that there are many nurturing styles, most specialists concur on some broad rules for supporting a kid's enthusiastic wellbeing and laying the preparation for a genuinely sound adulthood.

Know about stages in kid advancement so you don't expect excessively or excessively little from your youngster.

Urge your kid to communicate their sentiments; regard those emotions. Tell your kid that everybody encounters torment, dread, outrage, and tension. Attempt to get familiar with the wellspring of these sentiments. Help your youngster express displeasure decidedly, without falling back on savagery.

Advance common regard and trust. Keep your voice level down — in any event, when you disagree. Keep correspondence channels open.

Tune in to your youngster. Use words and models your youngster can comprehend. Empower questions. Give solace and confirmation. Be straightforward. Zero in on the positives. Express your ability to discuss any subject.

Take a gander at your own critical thinking and adapting abilities. Is it accurate to say that you are setting a genuine model? Look for help in the event that you are overpowered by your kid's sentiments or practices, or on the off chance that you can't handle your own dissatisfaction or outrage.

Empower your youngster's abilities and acknowledge restrictions. Put forward objectives dependent on the kid's capacities and interests — not another person's assumptions. Commend achievements. Try not to contrast your youngster's capacities with those of different kids; appreciate the uniqueness of your kid. Invest energy routinely with your youngster.

Cultivate your kid's autonomy and self-esteem. Help your youngster manage life's good and bad times. Show trust in your kid's capacity to deal with issues and tackle new encounters.

Control valuably, decently, and reliably. Use discipline as a type of instructing, not actual discipline. All youngsters and families are extraordinary; realize what is compelling for your kid. Show endorsement for positive practices. Assist your kid with learning their mix-ups.

Love genuinely. Show the worth of conciliatory sentiments, participation, persistence, absolution, and thought for other people.

Try not to hope to be awesome; nurturing is a troublesome work.

Chapter 3

Eight different ways to support a Kid's spirit

I am a nurturer of spirits, as are you.

We mothers (and truly, all individuals) have the chance to impact the spirits of the youngsters in our consideration. It can feel overpowering, simply pondering what that implies; that we are fit for developing an entire life, starting in the inward most pieces of a being. It's faltering, truly, what we are prepared to do in the event that we are purposeful and cherishing.

In contemplating the meaning of our impact, I'd prefer to offer a couple of ways you can sustain a youngster's spirit.

Be a sorter of their knot.

How delicate is a youthful heart, and how effectively wounds putrefy. I'm 22 and I marvel at the injuries in my own heart. I feel more unwound now than any time in recent memory; opportunity is all over me since I have understanding – I've lived and I've battled for opportunity.

My little ones, they don't comprehend the totality of absolution and brokenness and agony and shamefulness. They haven't lived enough. It's mistaking for them; they simply know how they feel. I'm the sorter-external.

We, us mothers and daddies, we're the ones who need to keep at the arranging. We should continue tuning in, truly tuning in, knowing, and encouraging our darlings so they can be available to opportunity. With empathy, persistence, and time we offer ourselves to crafted by arranging the heart strings so one day they'll be available to having them tied up new and excellent.

Cause them to feel like the main individual on the planet.

Our kids, actually like us, need to be known. They need to be regarded. They need to realize they matter more than any other individual, since they are our own.

Take the time from time to time to give them your complete consideration. Give them your arms to incline toward. Give them your eyes and your grin. Cause them to feel like the main individual on the planet.

Since at this time, they are particle to not satisfy you.

Your youngsters are made extraordinarily and perfectly, and they have sentiments and tastes that frequently will be inverse from your own. Acknowledge it, and permit them to be free in what their identity is.

Tell them that they are not liable for satisfying you. Tell them that they fulfill you since they're yours. Allow them to not satisfy you. It's a liberating thing.

Regard them.

I accept that regarding our youngsters is absolutely critical. I need my kids to realize that when they say "no" or "stop" that they ought to be tuned in to, regarded. In case I'm stimulating my darlings and they say stop, I stop. On the off chance that I go to rub their back and they say stop, I stop (and I don't cause them to feel remorseful for it).

We ought not be insulted if our kids don't want to embrace, or being tickled, or getting it done, or whatever. They are developing into what their identity is and what they like and don't care for, and we need to regard their limits, similarly as we need our limits regarded.

They need to realize that what they say matters, that we care about their conclusions and emotions and bents. It's not just how we regard them; it's the means by which we acquire their trust. What's more, I need the trust of my youngsters. I bet you do, as well.

We should tune in to our angels and offer them a protected spot to develop and learn and extend into what their identity is. How about we regard those little loves of our own?

Be their closest companion.

Gracious, how frequently I have heard, "You are not your kid's companion, you are their parent."

I'm my kid's parent, this is valid, but on the other hand I'm attempting to be her companion. I'm attempting to develop our relationship now by tolerating her, showing her beauty, showing her, cherishing her well, tuning in to her, viewing her appropriately, being straightforward with her, and regarding her. My "work" as a parent is to assist her figure with trip the world, and to live well and to cherish others.

What's more, isn't it equivalent to a companion? To share and chuckle and gain from one another as we sort out coexistence? As we go through the good and bad times of regular, together? As we figure out how to cherish and pardon and incline toward truth, together?

Indeed, that is fellowship, and I trust and will be closest companions with my kid.

Talk benevolent to them.

On the off chance that you find that you are talking cruelly to your youngsters, or hollering at them to an extreme, or you end up letting completely go when you blow up, if it's not too much trouble, get on your knees and decide to change. Be defenseless, and don't surrender when the change doesn't occur right away.

Request that your kids pardon you, and disclose to them you are a wreck a few days (we as a whole are). Be straightforward with them; give them the regard that you would need. Or more all, don't get debilitate that you won't ever transform; you can transform, you do have authority over your indignation. Graciousness is a blessing you can give your kids. Unwrap constantly it.

Tell them disgrace isn't welcomed into your family.

Tell your kids that you won't ever teach them for disclosing to you something they should be liberated from. Tell them whatever it is, whatever yuck has occurred, whatever to anything, that they can confide in you. Tell them you are there for them, and you're in their group. Furthermore, would not joke about this.

Since disgrace says, "They'll be distraught at you, and they'll fault you, and you are appalling and terrible and it's all your issue in any case."

Disgrace is a liar when you know reality – reality that you are not your wreck or anybody else's. Reality that you can be free. Leave your youngsters alone allowed to be completely forthright with you, and ensure they realize they have your open arms.

Show them that you start once more.

We as a whole mess up, ordinary, however we don't need to remain there in the wreck. Indeed, we can, on the off chance that we decide to remain solidified, to not apologize, to not acknowledge effortlessness.

However, we additionally have the decision to lay ourselves low. We can feel distress and we can get up from the waste. We can go into genuine love when we break before others and permit ourselves to be recuperated; they see the retouching and the scars, however they pardon us, as we excuse them.

This is elegance and opportunity. What's more, with elegance and opportunity there is no space for strain – the excruciating, terrible pressure that chokes a spirit.

Nurturing heart

In the sustain job, you deal with your youngsters' essential requirements, like food, clinical consideration, cover, attire, and so on, just as give love, consideration, getting, acknowledgment, time, and backing.

You tune in to your youngsters, are patient, and mess around with them. You set aside a few minutes for your children, show an interest in them and their exercises, and urge them to seek after their interests. Through your words and activities, you convey to your youngsters that they are cherished and acknowledged.

At the point when you are in the supporting job, you appreciate and acknowledge your youngsters as they are and don't anticipate any adjustment of conduct.

The advantages of the Sustain Job

At the point when you are sustaining, your youngsters; have a positive outlook on themselves;feel adorable and deserving of being really focused on; feel tuned in to – become familiar with their thoughts, sentiments, and necessities are significant – and feel that they are perceived; become trusting in light of the fact that they realize that their necessities will be met.

Discover that they can handle tough spots and face difficulties since they don't need to confront them alone – you will be there to help them.

Can reward others through the passionate help they are given from you. This forms their capacity to understand others.

It is through adoring and strong early parent-youngster connections that the establishments for future solid connections are framed. Being esteemed only for whom they are assists with building your kid's confidence.

This is a vital piece of your nurturing position. It is this job that numerous individuals know instinctively is basic for their kids' sound turn of events.

What amount support to give?

The measure of parental consideration and contribution should be burdened a scale, as demonstrated beneath.

At the point when you give a lot sustain, you might be excessively defensive, excessively receptive to your kids' requirements, and too engaged with their lives.

Under these conditions, kids don't acquire abilities to really focus on themselves and they don't figure out how to consider others' requirements.

On the other hand, when you're not supporting enough, you are too genuinely removed and not satisfactorily associated with your kids' lives.

Subsequently, youngsters don't feel cherished or upheld and they don't figure out how to confide in others.

To an extreme or too little support

The Construction Job

Kid going through finish line The other aspect of your responsibilities as a parent is to give "structure" for your youngsters. In this job, you provide guidance, force rules, use discipline, put down certain boundaries, set up and finish results, consider your kids responsible for their conduct, and

Instruct values.

You give the direction that assists your youngsters with evolving, develop, and develop. Mindful conduct, in accordance with your youngsters' development levels, is instructed and anticipated. In the construction job, you anticipate change in conduct and expanded development, development, and capacity.

The advantages of the Construction Job

When giving construction, your Kids:

feel a feeling of wellbeing that rules will be set up when they can't handle their own motivations – you will be there to stop them, manage them, and be accountable for their prosperity.

Figure out how to endure a sensible measure of dissatisfaction and frustration when they don't generally get their own particular manner.

Find that the world doesn't rotate absolutely around them. Subsequently, they become less egocentric. Learn mindful conduct and that they can do things. Gain from their errors. Acquire experience deciding. Become more independent and able as they get familiar with the abilities to get autonomous.

Disguise your principles and qualities.

Frequently guardians have more trouble completing this capacity in a sound manner. However it is crucially critical to your youngsters' advancement that you discipline them, show them, control them, give manages and finish the guidelines, and set sensible assumptions for their conduct. You don't need to be mean as you put down certain boundaries.

For instance, in the event that you plunk down with your kid to set a timetable for extra-curricular exercises, you are giving direction. In the event that you have your child perused three pages of a book so anyone might hear to rehearse his perusing abilities which his instructor has said are underneath grade level, you would give structure.

It might in any case be a warm and adoring communication, yet you will likely assist your youngster with developing and procure new abilities; subsequently, you are giving design.

By holding youngsters to guidelines and assisting them with making progress, you assist them with feeling proficient and consequently fabricate their confidence.

What amount construction to give?

Very much like with the Sustain Job, the Design Job exists on a scale as demonstrated beneath.

At the point when you give a lot structure, you might be inflexible and utilize cruel control; kids don't figure out how to have an independent perspective, and they may either get aloof or they may revolt.

At the point when you give too little design, your assumptions and rules might be indistinct and conflicting. Kids may feel confounded; they don't feel that they will be ensured; and they don't figure out how to be dependable in light of the fact that they are not considered responsible for their practices.

Harmony between something over the top and too little design

Discovering the Harmony among Sustain and Design

As well as discovering a spot on every one of these two scales that dodges the limits of giving excessively or excessively minimal mindful or control, you likewise need to discover a harmony among how and when to sustain your youngsters and how and when to give structure.

With the goal for youngsters to flourish and create in a sound manner, they need you to do both of these jobs. The harmony between the two jobs that you accomplish has an effect.

In the event that you just give the support piece with no construction or limits or without considering kids responsible, your kids can get ruined, unappreciative, conceited, and not figure out how to get things done for themselves.

These are signs of an "indulged" youngster. Your youngsters may confuse your consideration with shortcoming and not view you as a wellspring of help.

In the event that you just give the design piece without building a solid relationship of trust, your kids may feel angry, disliked, deserted, and might be less inclined to collaborate readily with the guidelines or to disguise them.

Dreading discipline, kids may attempt to fly under the radar and conceal their errors and weaknesses from you. You will pass up on freedoms to impact your youngsters' practices and decisions.

Harmony among support and construction

Your kids need you to give both sustain and design. As you communicate with your kids, deliberately choose if you need to give more love and consideration or in the event that you need to give more design and direction.

Suppose your kid just tossed a ball in the house and broke a photo placement. Your first intuition might be to train him. Notwithstanding, on the off chance that he is actually harmed or terrified, you may conclude that you should support first and quiet your kid down before you talk about the need to tidy up the messed up glass and why you have a standard against ball-playing in the house in any case.

On the other hand, your little girl might resent her sibling who by and by acquired her school supplies and neglected to return them. This is an on-going grievance and you comprehend your little girl's dissatisfaction. Notwithstanding, her hitting her sibling is unsatisfactory and you may have to uphold the standard of "no hitting" before you assist her arrangement with her solid emotions.

There are no immovable principles about when you ought to sustain or when you should utilize structure. You may settle on one choice in one circumstance with one youngster and settle on an alternate decision at some other point. It is the general equilibrium that is significant and that impacts your youngsters' turn of events – not your decision at any one time.

The Effect of Your Youth

It very well may be useful to venture back and consider your own adolescence.

How very much did your folks balance the jobs of sustain and construction?

How does this contrast with your own nurturing inclination?

Frequently, if individuals were brought up in an excessively organized climate with severe and inflexible control set up, they may wind up avoiding such nurturing with their own youngsters and inclining too intensely on the supporting side of things.

And keeping in mind that it can feel better in the short-run for you to be the "pleasant person," it doesn't normally work out for you or your youngsters over the long haul.

For instance, after a long, warm, and debilitating summer day, your youngsters request that you take them out for frozen yogurt. All you need to do is sit in a decent cool room; yet being a "pleasant" parent, you concur and head out to the frozen yogurt parlor.

As a trade-off for your liberality, you expect the least your children could do isn't battle with each other or protest at you when you berate them to turn the television and clean up.

However, they do battle with each other and you. You may get angry – all things considered, you made a special effort to be "pleasant."

What's going on with them? Now you may "explode" and turn into that excessively forceful parent that you were making a decent attempt to abstain from being in any case.

Chapter 4

Co-Nurturing

It can likewise be useful to consider what inclinations you and any co-guardians have toward giving more support or more design. This is regularly affected by how every one of you was raised.

It is regular for guardians to move in various ways after some time because of the other parent's methodology. Here is the means by which this can work:

Parent Support normally inclines toward being really sustaining, while Parent Design is slanted toward giving construction.

Over the long run, Parent Design may think Parent Support has been too simple on the youngster and that the kid isn't tuning in to asks for, is acting ruined, and donning an "disposition." accordingly, Parent Construction sets some hard boundaries and advises the kid he is relied upon to observe the principles.

Parent Support thinks Parent Construction is excessively brutal and not comprehension of the kid. To help the youngster feel good, Parent Support goes simpler on the kid when they are together. Parent Construction, seeing no improvement in conduct, turns out to be much stricter. Parent Support turns out to be significantly more remiss with less prerequisites on the kid.

This can proceed until one parent turns into the sole drill sergeant and the other is the sole nurturer.

This set-up isn't to the greatest advantage of you, your youngster or your co-parent. It sets up power battles among guardians and can empower your youngsters to control you.

While each parent may have their regular inclinations toward the support or design side of things, preferably, both you and your co-parent will actually want to comfort your kid and give direction.

Finding some kind of harmony is a test and adds to making nurturing a workmanship as opposed to a science.

In Synopsis

While the occasions to sustain and the occasions to give construction will fluctuate dependent on the kid, the conditions, and the guardians, it assists with making a stride back and intentionally choose in a specific circumstance what job will best assist your kid with developing and learn – the support job or the design job.

All in all, it is a combination of both inclusion and control that will assist your kids with getting the inner assets they should succeed.

It is actually a debilitating, confounded, yet remunerating position to parent your kids and fulfill their vital requirements.

The Sustaining Guardian

Misuse, disregard, relinquishment, brutality and kidnapping ... these terrible truths are what numerous youngsters in America live with. Tragically, viciousness and disregard towards kids is the same old thing ... it is profoundly established in social and strict qualities.

We should support our kids ...it is one of the significant things we can do. A guardian's adoration and caring decides how a youngster grows up and how a kid will in the end parent.

Grown-ups can support youngsters' positive confidence by assisting them with finding what they are acceptable at doing. Some portion of a kid's confidence comes from feeling capable and gifted at something they appreciate. By setting out open doors for youngsters to investigate various articles, exercises, and individuals ... what's more, sustaining those interests, you can assume a major part in assisting youngsters with being fruitful and have a positive outlook on themselves.

The early years are when kids show character qualities and inclinations for what they like and abhorrence. By arranging openings in light of youngsters' exceptional character styles, you sustain their good emotions about themselves.

Supporting youngsters, constructing an adoring and caring relationship isn't in every case simple. With tolerance and love – you can do it!

Treat every youngster as indicated by their requirements.

Each youngster needs guardians who can see and like their unique characteristics. At the point when kin are included, attempting to treat each similarly generally misfires and subverts kids' singularity.

Center consideration at whatever point conceivable, keeping away from interruptions

In the event that youngsters need to associate when you can't be completely mindful, let them know and timetable a period for discussion or potentially play when you can zero in altogether on them. Kids generally know when grown-ups are just half-tuning in and can feel disappointed, unheard, and on occasion even dislike when this occurs. Tuning in to kids with your complete consideration reinforces their feeling of significance and gives the message that you truly need to hear their opinion and feeling.

Listen delicately, keep away from (something over the top) addressing, and depict the circumstance.

Kids will normally close down genuinely when guardians assault them with questions. They feel on the spot and constrained when grown-ups test and ask a lot about their day. Depicting the circumstance is a nonpartisan and non-meddling methodology that leaves space for youngsters to react in their own particular manner.

Use "I" messages and attempt to abstain from accusing and allegations. This will permit you to communicate your sentiments about a specific conduct without assaulting your kid's character or confidence.

Put down certain boundaries that are proper to youngsters' age, disposition and phase of improvement.

At the point when guardians have restricted time with their youngsters, they may will in general release things and not put forth sensible and fundamental lines. Youngsters need to realize that you – their parent or guardian have the interest, energy and power to set suitable principles for conduct and the abilities to finish.

Start customs that vibe agreeable and fit your nurturing style and monetary assets. Customs furnish kids with a significant feeling of having a place. They don't need to be intricate to be fun or essential. The main thing you can do to begin another practice (or proceed with an old one) is whatever feels great and charming for both the guardians and kids. Customs are additionally significant for showing kids - and focusing them in their societies.

Deal with yourself so you have energy and eagerness accessible for your youngsters. It very well may be elusive a harmony between addressing your youngsters' necessities and setting aside a few minutes for yourselves. It is significant for you to discover proper source for your sensations of stress, obligations, and so forth, and you need some 'down' an ideal opportunity to seek after your own advantages or just to loosen up. Most guardians track down that even a brief break from kids can have a constructive outcome in the manner they feel.

Guardians need to satisfy themselves as guardians, in their nurturing jobs, and furthermore as people with interests outside the family. They need to go spots all alone, and to do a few things only for themselves. At that point guardians get back to their kids invigorated.

At the point when you're pushed:

Attempt to determine circumstances before they heighten.

Invest some energy.

Call somebody and express how you're feeling. Request that they come over and stay with the children for some time.

Recollect the amount you love your kid and consider the most ideal approach to show that to your youngster.

Protect your youngsters, regardless!

The most ideal approach to protect kids is to hold them back from getting injured in any case. Numerous guardians who do make hurt their youngsters don't mean

to do it. In the event that a parent was disregarded or mishandled as a kid, it is possible that a lot harder to change to a more helpful conduct with their own children. There is a plenitude of help and data accessible to assist guardians with achieving bringing up sound and safe youngsters. There are numerous approaches to effectively deal with a kid's conduct. At the point when grown-ups figure out how to depend on useful, non-terrible nurturing, both parent and kid rest easy thinking about themselves. Positive nurturing approaches assist the entire family with flourishing. These methodologies can be seen in different parts of their lives also. Guardians even accomplish better busy working and their youngsters are more effective in school.

There are two kinds of youth encounters:

Positive encounters; that form solid character and an ability to be self aware worth that model a sustaining nurturing style.

Negative encounters; that immerse youngsters in nurturing models of misuse, disregard, abuse, and exploitation.

The best nurturing comes from guardians who establish a climate that produces encounters that influence the development of the individual kid. The supporting guardian utilizes a sustaining contact, sympathy, strengthening, and unequivocal love to guarantee the general wellbeing of their kid.

Oppressive guardians who use hitting, deprecating, disregarding fundamental requirements, and different activities that bring down a person's self-appreciation worth ...or more awful, have a pessimistic effect on the wellbeing of their youngster.

Kid misuse has an impeding effect on a kid's mental self portrait, giving them sensations of low confidence, which impacts how they will treat others. Youngsters who esteem themselves and approach themselves with deference show a similar conduct toward others. The association between self-esteem and the value of others is basic in kid misuse avoidance. Sustaining has been demonstrated to be a positive effect on a youngster's mental self portrait and self-esteem.

Kid misuse is the aftereffect of ineffectively prepared grown-ups who as guardians and parental figures, attempt to impart teach and instruct youngsters with the very brutality that they, at the end of the day, experienced as kids ...since that is all they know.

Nurturing is learned in adolescence and rehashed when kids become guardians. The encounters youngsters have while growing up, have a critical effect on the mentalities, abilities, and nurturing rehearses they will use with their own kids.

What is realized can be untaught and anybody and everybody can master great nurturing abilities. Indeed, even guardians who are overpowered, or alone. The initial three years of your youngster's life are pivotal. Those are the years that your youngster will create huge scholarly, enthusiastic and social capacities. That is the point at which they figure out how to give and acknowledge love. They learn certainty, security, and sympathy ... they figure out how to be interested and relentless ... all your kid requires to figure out how to relate well to other people, and lead a glad and profitable life. The initial three years are the entryway to for eternity!

Sustaining youngsters is about the manner in which we love them ...the manner in which we bring them up. A parent's adoration is our youngsters' fate. It's the heritage we give them.

What is a Supporting Relationship and How to Look after It?

A supporting relationship for adolescents is a blend and utilization of many fitting guardian/kid co operations and practices. There are numerous contemplations on the legitimate nurturing procedures for the pre-teenager kids. Dr. Phil has his, Mother has hers, Dr. Ruth has hers, etc! The Supporting Relationship Program that I advance in this book is a blend of numerous uplifting feedback strategies alongside a sustaining demeanor to improve legitimate control and conduct. I don't advance any sort of physical or mental maltreatment like hitting and hollering. You may say that I was hit and I ended up good overall. All things considered, I was additionally punished and I turned out truly well, yet I trusted I was disabled in my initial a long time from an absence of confidence and being modest. Through relentlessness and tirelessness I had the option to beat a portion of these impairments, albeit a portion of these shortcomings actually frequent me today. I accept that in the event that I had a Sustaining Relationship with my folks, large numbers of these shortcomings would not be available in my initial years and my life would have less unrest.

What is supporting?

Sustaining is a basic expertise for all life structures on the planet. For people, it is maybe the absolute most significant trademark to have for us all to live in harmony, bliss and serenity. When sustaining is absent, clearly individuals can be noxious and appalling to one another. How does supporting affect us?

To observe the Brilliant Standard, which is "treat others the manner in which you need to be dealt with yourself."

Regard and care for yourself, others and the climate.

Try not to hurt yourself, others or the climate.

Realize that everything around you have worth and worth.

There is acceptable in every way.

Having a sustaining connection with your youngster is to bring your kid up in a mindful, cherishing, trusting and vehement home. The are a few things that advance a supporting relationship.

Correspondence - It is imperative to permit youngsters to communicate their sentiments and to approve their emotions. Very much like grown-ups, youngsters are anxious to discuss the things that occurred during their day and to communicate the genuine emotions about something. The kid can be pitiful or baffled and it is significant that parent knows this. The parent ought to consistently tune in to what the kid says and pose great inquiries, if fundamental.

Figuring out how to stroll from someone else's point of view is called Sympathy, which is the one most alluring quality in supporting connections. Compassion is the capacity to know about the requirements of others and comprehend the significance of those necessities. At the point when compassion is high among relatives, misuse is commonly low—the two are practically contradictory. The Supporting Relationship Program looks to create sympathy in all relatives through common regard and correspondence.

Figure out how to Support Yourself - You can't sustain others on the off chance that you are drained and angry that they are getting the entirety of the adoration and consideration. To defeat these emotions you should sustain yourself in any event once every day. For instance, on your path home from work require 10 minutes and pass by and get a frozen treat at Baskin and Robbins that you can appreciate in transit home. Peruse a book. Go for a short stroll with a companion or without anyone else. Do a few activities. Simply invest some energy just for you. In the event that you consistently penance your requirements for the necessities of others, you will wear out and be vexed and furious more often than not. 10-15 minutes daily can mean a ton for your prosperity so take care of business!

Really focusing on Youngsters Utilizing Delicate Embraces and Contact - You can convey to the kid through an embrace or delicate intense that you give it a second thought and love them. Delicate touch has been read for generations. Delicate touch and embraces show the kid you give it a second thought and it causes them to feel exceptional. Appearing and telling the kid that you care for them and love them expands their self-esteem. Where and when loves start for the youngster. Some say, love begins with the guardians before birth when they intellectually plan to put the child in their souls and lives. Others say the primary love is the point at which they see the child interestingly. From a characteristic human propensity, love and sustaining is grown normally during the baby long stretches of the youngster and as a rule proceeds for the remainder of their lives.

Say that you care for them and Love them consistently. You may say that they definitely know this, however they don't. By revealing to them this at the correct time, they feel an incredible fulfillment that their folks truly care and love them. Tell them this is unequivocal love and you love them only for what their identity is. Never present and partner love with errands, for example, "I love you for tidying up your room". This isn't unrestricted love - it was contingent dependent on tidying up your room. Say, when you are have a straightforward discussion with the youngster, "And something other, Jason, I love you for what your identity is and I generally will adore you regardless of what occurs in our coexistences"

Order is significant for the youngster's soundness. Youngsters are searching for a climate that has structure and where they realize what's in store. Too often guardians are not reliable is restraining the kid and the youngster is truly confounded on what is correct and what's up. It is critical to set up decides for the family that are applied in a steady way with set up ramifications for keeping or disrupting the guidelines. Building up family runs is a vital piece of the supporting relationship program and will be examined in a later section.

Throughout the long term, guardians hear numerous things about fruitful nurturing and how to achieve it viably. A significant number of these methodologies are not in accordance with building up a supporting relationship. A portion of the methodologies and truisms from guardians that I hear consistently are "My Direction or the Roadway", "This will hurt me more than it will hurt you", "One Day You'll Express gratitude toward Me", "The Book of scriptures Says to Do It That Way!", the "Alright Methodology" and "Embrace Them and Snuggle Them". As I would like to think, these are an alternate ways to nurturing. Each can be performed quickly and has next to no advantageous long haul impact.

The "My Way or the Parkway" approach implies exactly what it says. You as the parent is in finished charge of the house and world where the family resides and if the youngster doesn't care for the manner in which we are doing it the kid can leave or be squashed. This was an incredible way of thinking for Attila the Hun and Adolf Hitler, yet for creating youthful personalities to coexist with others and to have extraordinary connections, and this despot approach doesn't work.

The "This Will Hurt Me More Than It Will Hurt You" is only a pardon to beat on the kid, accepting that the youngster thinks you are truly wish you didn't need to do that. Truly, doubtlessly, the parent has let completely go with outrage from something that happened before in the day and has hit the kid over and again because of some minor offense that the kid has made. Presently do you truly accept the kid thinks this damages the parent more than the one being beaten?

I like the one where the parent says "One Day You'll Say thanks to me". The parent that expresses this crazy assertion accepts that this actual maltreatment, for example, hitting will assist the kid with being a superior individual later on and ,around then later on, the kid turned grown-up will thank the parent for every one of the beatings that where directed while the person in question was growing up. This is, obviously, is irrational. I can't think about any beating, which my mom or father gave as direction to me, that I needed to express gratitude toward them for the magnificent and caring direction

In the event that you take a gander at what Jesus did during his life on earth, there was consistently a unique spot in His heart for the youngsters. Hitting is contrary to the Brilliant Guideline, which is the main principle that Jesus gave us for human relationships. The Brilliant Principle is " treat others the manner in which you need to be dealt with yourself." And apparently we would prefer not to be hit or beaten in any capacity, so we shouldn't hit others, and since youngsters are individuals, clearly we shouldn't do that to kids. The brilliant guideline is embraced by every one of the incredible world religions; Jesus, Hillel, and Confucius utilized it to sum up their moral lessons, and for a long time the thought has been powerful among individuals of different societies. These realities propose that the brilliant guideline might be a significant good truth. This implies that the ethical truth for the total populace is to not hit or beat your kids!

The "Alright Methodology" We are going to Auntie Ann's home now, alright. We are going to tidy up our room now, alright. We won't lie any longer, take medications, or take from K-Store, alright. I realize it could be a propensity, yet when guardians inquire as to whether it is alright to accomplish something that they need to do, it makes them look senseless. Asking youngsters is it alright for them to go along or show appropriate conduct. Crazy!! You ought to anticipate consistence and appropriate conduct from your youngsters. We are going to Auntie Ann's home in a short time, and I anticipate that you should have your shoes and socks on and in vehicle when we are prepared to leave. Large distinction between requesting consistence and anticipating consistence. Along these lines, we will fail to remember the alright methodology, alright!

"Embrace them and Snuggle Them" is performed by a parent who truly cares and loves their kids, however this is the limit inverse to manhandle despite the fact that it is really not useful for the kid. On the off chance that you are embracing them and snuggling them the entirety of the time you truly don't possess any energy for supporter. Devotee is critical in a youngster's life. It gives design and consistency that is fundamental for a solid confidence should have been fruitful throughout everyday life. It is essential to embrace and nestle them now and again, however just low maintenance. The other part ought to be tied in with figuring out how to act naturally adequate and building up a decent self idea, which must be accomplished with self inspired youngsters and adoring and caring guardians that show them the way.

Great nurturing is a troublesome and tedious occupation for a parent, however the prizes are very satisfying when you see your youngsters grow up to be certain and independent grown-ups. One of the main territories that should be created in a supporting relationship is the family runs the show.

Family Practice Exercise (30-45 minutes)

Get along with your close family. This is essentially individuals who live in your family. Attempt to get everybody there possibly just after supper. Structure a little circle sitting in seats (This could be during supper) or on the floor (perhaps in the living or family room). Have them perused the past segment about sustaining connections or read it to them.

Character and Good Knowledge, Nurturing

In spite of the fact that most educators concede that there are a few understudies they always remember, the equivalent is valid about guardians.

I clearly recall a mother of one of my understudies all due to the manner in which she passed on regard to her kid. She did so wonderfully by them way she tuned in. I watched her multiple times over time on our field trips and in our group parties or simply those occasions she'd stand by at the way to get him. Each time Ricky would talk, she'd stop what she'd do, get down to eye level, investigate her child's eyes, and tune in with authentic premium. She had this superb capacity to shut out everything–or possibly cause her youngster to feel she was–and give her kid her full presence. The time was brief – one moment or somewhere in the vicinity.

The mother's words ordinarily were just rehashing back little goodies of what he just said just to tell him she was hearing him. Sometimes she'd add, "Uh-huh," or "Truly?" She recognized him just by saying how she thought he was feeling: "You appear to be so glad" or "Goodness, you look pleased."

The impact on her child was sensational: Ricky's entire attitude lit up when he understood his mother sincerely heard what he needed to say. I generally wished I might have recorded her listening abilities to play back to different guardians. The mother's practices were so straightforward, yet consistently passed on regard to her kid. That mother exemplified perhaps the most impressive, dependable character-building rehearses there is: "The most ideal approach to guarantee that our children are conscious is to treat them deferentially."

It should not shock anyone that her youngster ended up being one of my most aware understudies. He additionally developed to turn into a deferential grown-up.

That is a direct result of this significant standard: youngsters gain regard best from seeing and encountering regard.

So Mother and Father: Tune up regard in your own conduct. All things considered, it's a scandalous, uncivilized world out there. I dread what our children are seeing and encountering slight.

Seven Straightforward Regard Building Nurturing Practices

Here are seven straightforward nurturing rehearses that help kids consider themselves to be important individuals. The practices work to ingrain regard in your kid all in light of the fact that your activities let them realize you love, regard, and worth them. Your kid is likewise seeing and encountering regard with these practices so he is bound to embrace and utilize the excellence.

1. Treat your kid as the main individual on the planet.

Here is a straightforward inquiry to pose to yourself: "On the off chance that I treated my companions the manner in which I treat my youngster, how might my companions react?" (Or would you have any companions left? Well) Be careful: all the time we say and get things done to our kids that our companions could never endure.

In the event that you need your kids to feel esteemed, treat them like they are the main individuals on the planet. One mother revealed to me she asked herself the inquiry so frequently it turned into an evening time propensity. It likewise assisted her with recollecting the day to treat her youngsters deferentially.

2. Give love without any hidden obligations.

No kid ought to need to procure our regard and love; it ought to be ensured with birth. Unlimited love is tied in with cherishing your children without any surprises. It is the sort of adoration that says: "I'll love constantly you regardless of what you do." obviously, that doesn't mean we will fundamentally favor the entirety of our kids' practices. At times when our children's activities are unseemly we may have to react with clear and frequently energetic amendment. Yet, our children realize we'll generally be there for them-regardless and that is the sort of affection our children need on the off chance that they are to feel they are truly regarded and esteemed. Ensure you give your youngster love that is genuine and ensured so regardless of what he realizes you love him.

3. Listen mindfully and consciously.

On the off chance that there is one basic finding from innumerable various investigations it is that children say they wish their folks would listen-truly hear them out. Mindful listening is a great method to pass on regard.

At the point when your kid talks, quit everything and concentrate totally with the goal that she feels you truly esteem her sentiments and need to hear her musings. Stop what you're doing and give your kid your full presence for the short time.

Clue: Juvenile young men are regularly undermined by eye to eye connection, so have a go at sitting side to side.

4. Discuss regard with your entire body, not simply with your words.

More often than not our children aren't tuning in to our words close to however much they are watching our stance, signals, and looks and hearing our manner of speaking. So ensure your entire body is conveying regard when you converse with your youngster. You may say, "I need to hear your thoughts," yet on the off chance that your kid sees you shrug your shoulders, raise your eye temples, grins your mouth, or feign exacerbation; he is probably going to get an entire diverse importance.

I've yet to meet guardians who need their children to figure they aren't keen on their thoughts or don't regard their children's emotions. However those are the messages kids get, all as a result of how guardians respond when their youngsters talk.

5. Assemble positive self-ideas.

Marking youngsters with so much terms as timid, difficult, hyper, or cumbersome can decrease confidence and become every day tokens of disgracefulness. They can likewise become unavoidable outcomes.

Whether or not the names are valid or not, when youngsters hear them they trust them. So just use names that form positive self-ideas. One great principle to recollect about marking is this: "If the moniker isn't deferential, it's best not to utilize it."

6. Explain to them regularly why you adore and treasure them.

The more you show your kid you love her, the more your youngster figures out how to esteem and cherish herself. So tell your youngster frequently that you love her, yet additionally mention to her what you love about her and offer your thanks that she is your kid.

I love that you are so kind. I'm so happy I have the fortune of being your mother. I love you simply the manner in which you are. I regard the manner in which you won't ever surrender.

Never accept that your youngster understands what sentiments you hold in your heart about her. Advise her.

7. Partake in being together.

Probably the most ideal approaches to help a youngster feel regarded is to tell her the amount you appreciate being with her. Put your youngster at the highest point of your timetable and put away loosened up occasions together during which you can truly become more acquainted with who your kid is. Really at that time can you let her know why you worth, love, and regard her so.

A fast test is to ask yourself which attributes you regard in your youngster. Would your youngster have the option to name those qualities also?

So now the genuine nurturing test: Recall throughout the most recent couple of days. What have you done that helps your youngsters consider themselves to be important people in light of the fact that your activities let them realize you love, regard, and worth them? Remember that our basic everyday activities are regularly the most impressive approaches to support regard in our youngsters.

CHAPTER 5

CONCLUSION

Let remember that nurturing implies more than giving your kid food, haven and attire. It is tied in with building a solid and forceful enthusiastic relationship (connection) among you and your kid. And a proper understanding of the sub-topics will actually emancipate any parent who long to properly nurture his or her kid. Our nation will be great again when our children are properly and deliberate nurtured.

In addition nurturing is learned in adolescence and rehashed when kids become guardians. The encounters youngsters have while growing up, have a critical effect on the mentalities, abilities, and nurturing rehearses they will use with their own kids.